ATLAS OF BREAST EXAMINATION

2 JUN 2000			
20. MAY 2002			
20. MAY 2002			
15 AUG 2003			
24 JUN 2005			
27. MAY 2009			
3 0 OCT 2013			
22nd Nov			

ATLAS OF BREAST EXAMINATION

Ian S Fentiman and Hisham Hamed

ICRF Clinical Oncology Unit
Guy's Hospital
London, UK

Publishing
Group

© BMJ Publishing Group 1997

First published in 1997
by the BMJ Publishing Group, BMA House, Tavistock Square, London
WC1H 9JR

British Library Cataloguing in Publication Data

A catalogue record for this book is available from the British Library

ISBN 0–7279–0857–X

Typeset by Apek Typesetters Ltd, Nailsea, Bristol.
Printed and bound by Craft Print Plc Ltd, Singapore

CONTENTS

PREFACE   vii

1   GENERAL EXAMINATION   1

2   NIPPLES   8

3   NIPPLE DISCHARGE   16

4   BREAST PAIN   22

5   BREAST LUMPS IN YOUNG WOMEN   27

6   BREAST LUMPS IN MIDDLE-AGED WOMEN   32

7   BREAST LUMPS IN OLDER WOMEN   38

8   SKIN   45

9   BREAST CANCER   55

10 BREAST CANCER FOLLOW UP   59

    INDEX   67

PREFACE

We live in exciting and difficult times. The enormous investment which has been made in molecular biology is bearing fruit in terms of our understanding of breast cancer and the ability to detect individuals at risk.

Intense media interest in the field of breast cancer means that the public are aware of potential improvements and also learn about the treatment lottery. It is to be hoped that management will improve as quality assurance is introduced as an intrinsic part of the National Breast Cancer Screening Programme. Lurking behind the difficulties is the spectre of delayed diagnosis of breast cancer with attendant fears about litigation.

There is an apparently inexhaustible supply of worried women, spurred on by what they read, watch or hear from their peers. The first in line to receive these anxious patients are general practitioners and practice nurses, some of whom may have received training in breast examination and have the necessary communicational skills to reassure the majority of their patients and to detect the few with abnormalities who require specialist referral.

Others may be less than happy to deal with symptomatic women with breast problems. It is at them that this book is aimed. It does not undertake to be a comprehensive textbook of breast diseases. It is a window looking onto the field of breast cancer giving some practical advice on breast evaluation, and indicating some of the pitfalls.

The intention has been to illustrate the salient points of examination, and the commoner forms of breast pathology. We thank all of our patients who generously allowed us to photograph them and form the visual basis of this book.

ISF
HH

1
GENERAL EXAMINATION

The aim of breast examination is to detect those patients who have abnormalities requiring further assessment and, in the majority of cases, to reassure worried women with breast problems that they have no pathology. In order to give effective reassurance the patient must feel that her problem has been listened to with sympathy, and that a good clinical examination has been performed with an adequate and understandable explanation of the situation.

When any of these steps are omitted, patient anxiety or dissatisfaction can occur giving rise to long-term worry. Thus, if clinical breast examination has been effective a substantial number of unnecessary hospital referrals will be avoided. Additionally, a few women with small but significant breast lesions will be identified. Early diagnosis of breast cancers means that less extensive surgery will be required with a greater chance of cure.

History taking

The commonest breast symptom in general practice is pain, with or without associated lumpiness. It is important to ask whether this pain is cyclical or non-cyclical, localised or diffuse, and to what extent it interferes with the patient's life. Finding out whether the patient is worried about an underlying cancer, or is wanting treatment for the pain, is very important in further management. Often a patient will complain of a lump which proves, on subsequent examination, to be a localised area of nodularity, or part of a more widespread lumpiness.

Nipple discharge may be unilateral or bilateral, spontaneous or non-spontaneous. Further evaluation is needed in those with blood-containing discharge emerging from a single duct. Less common symptoms include nipple inversion and eczematous skin changes on or around the nipple–areolar complex.

1

Position of patient on couch

It is important that the patient is as comfortable as possible and caused minimal embarrassment during the examination. The patient can be examined either in the supine position or with the upper trunk at 45 degrees. The room and the examiner's hands should be warm. Good illumination is essential. Subtle changes may be missed in poor light. The patient should be asked to undress down to the waist, once a full history has been taken. Firstly, the breasts should be inspected with the arms by the side and note taken of asymmetry and changes in shape, together with abnormalities of the nipples and skin.

Elevation of arms

After inspection, the patient is asked to lift her hands above her head. This will demonstrate any limitation of shoulder movement, which may be part of a musculoskeletal condition giving rise to unilateral breast pain. Furthermore, arm elevation may bring the examiner's attention to skin dimpling caused by an underlying carcinoma, which may not be visible when the arms are by the side. In addition, this manoeuvre may reveal abnormalities in the inferior aspect of the breasts and the inframammary groove.

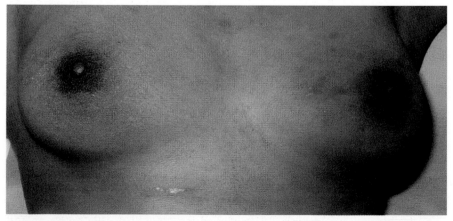

Figure 1.1
Inspection of normal breasts with arms elevated.

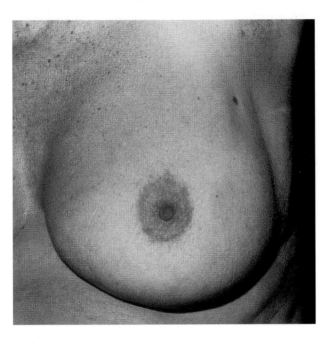

Figure 1.2
Skin dimpling seen only on elevation of the arm.

Demonstration of skin dimpling

Skin dimpling may be the symptom of which the patient complained, but more frequently it is a sign elicited during the examination and sometimes amplified on arm elevation. In patients with cancer, infiltration and fibrosis of the ligaments of Astley Cooper can produce either permanent skin puckering or dimpling on movement. However, although this can be a grave sign, it may result from prior surgery, fat necrosis, or localised superficial thrombophlebitis of a lateral thoracic vein (Mondor's syndrome).

Inspection with arms by the side

After the arms are placed by the patient's sides, a second inspection of the breasts can be conducted. In particular any areas which appeared abnormal previously should be checked, and it should be ascertained whether there is any residual skin dimpling or evidence of skin oedema (*peau d'orange*). Note is also taken of other signs which may give clues about the patient's personality and lifestyle – tattoos, bites, and needle tracks. Finally, prior surgical scars

3

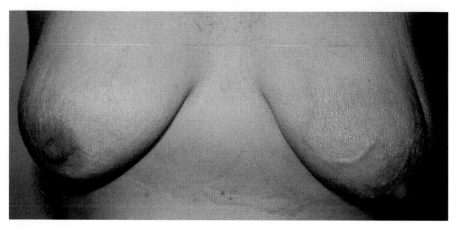

Figure 1.3
A case of Mondor's syndrome. Notice the characteristic longitudinal dimpling of the skin.

are sought and the patient questioned about the nature of the operation and histology, although most patients will know only that the lump was benign or 'just a piece of fatty tissue'.

Assessment of asymmetry

Some degree of asymmetry is very common and usually the left breast is slightly larger than the right. What is important is a recent change, with either increased growth on one side or, sometimes, shrinkage on the other. Similarly, unilateral nipple inversion which is longstanding is almost never of significance. Recent inversion with or without an associated lump does require further evaluation. Other features of asymmetry include differences in nipple height/position and the presence of accessory breast tissue in the milk line, extending from the axilla to the inguinal region.

Inspection of nipples

Shape, size, and colour of the nipples and areolae are noted, particularly when there is asymmetry. The accessory areolar glands of Montgomery are inspected and any cystic enlargement noted. Crusting, discharge, and eczematous change are sought.

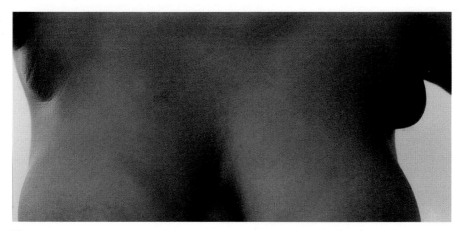

Figure 1.4

A case of bilateral axillary mammary gland. This condition is seen more commonly in black women.

When there is nipple indrawing this may be associated with a transverse slit, and this is usually pathognomic of duct ectasia giving rise to dilatation and shortening of the ducts, often associated with a nipple discharge. If an area of apparent eczema is seen on the nipple the patient should be asked whether she has any other eczematous patches. If not this increases suspicion of underlying malignancy. However, in any case this requires further evaluation to exclude Paget's disease of the nipple.

Palpation of the breasts

The most important aspect of breast examination is to carry out a methodical palpation so that all of the breast tissue has been checked. Additionally, when the patient has complained of a lump the examiner must convince her that the lesion has been carefully assessed. The patient is asked to point with a finger to the lump, if necessary sitting up since many women will state that they are able to find the lump only when in that position. The first breast that should be examined is the asymptomatic one, in order that attention is not distracted from contralateral pathology by the findings in the symptomatic breast.

Whether the examination is carried out with the flat of the hand or the tips of the fingers is unimportant. What matters is that a slow, careful and full check is carried out, either working up and down vertically or obliquely. This

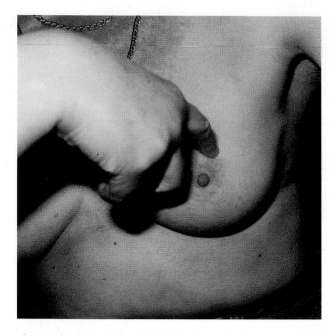

Figure 1.5
A patient pointing to
the site of the lump.
It was found to be
part of generalised
lumpiness.

is particularly difficult in fuller-breasted women. If this palpation is too hurried
the patient will not be convinced that it has been adequate and may demand
an unnecessary hospital referral or further hospital visits.

Inspection in the semilateral position

Once the breasts have both been examined with the patient lying on her
back, she is asked to turn half on her side either towards or away from the
examiner. She is asked to place her arm above her head. This manoeuvre
makes it possible to examine more thoroughly the upper outer quadrant,
axillary tail and axilla. The examiner re-palpates the breast obliquely so that
the upper outer quadrant which contains the bulk of the breast tissue has
been checked.

Palpation of axilla

Examination of the axilla is notoriously inaccurate, with great interobserver

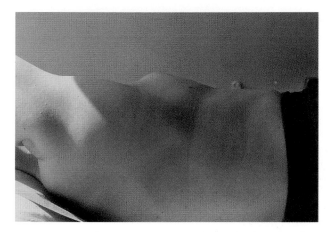

Figure 1.6
A patient in the left semilateral position. Note that a cystic lesion became more apparent once the patient was put in this position.

variation. In patients with breast cancer, approximately one-third who are deemed clinically to have no axillary nodal involvement will prove to have pathological involvement and one-third of those with palpable nodes will not have metastases.

Undoubtedly, axillary evaluation can be improved with experience. The most important part of the procedure is to relax the suspensory ligament of the axilla. This is done by palpating the axilla with the patient's arm by her side, supported by the examiner. If an attempt is made to examine the axilla with the shoulder abducted, this will result in inadequate evaluation.

KEY POINTS

- Most patients with breast symptoms require reassurance.
- Sympathetic history taking is essential.
- Careful and thorough examination is needed.
- Without taking the above steps, the patient will not be reassured.

2
NIPPLES

Normal

The normal virginal nipple is pink-brown and undergoes pigmentation during pregnancy and lactation. Between 10 and 15 accessory glands of Montgomery, which are cream-yellow in colour, are found in the nipple. The presence of hairs on the nipple is of no pathological consequence, although this may be more exaggerated in women with hirsutism due to excess androgens. A small amount of bilateral physiological nipple discharge is common and this may be milky in parous women. Mild galactorrhoea in women with regular menstrual cycles does not require investigation for hyperprolactinaemia. Pituitary adenomae secreting large amounts of

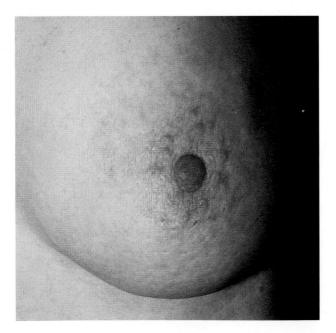

Figure 2.1

Normal nipple with Montgomery's glands.

prolactin give rise to irregular periods or amenorrhoea (galactorrhoea-amenorrhoea syndrome).

Montgomery's gland cyst

This may occur particularly in young women, and although it may cause great immediate concern, it usually resolves spontaneously. Only if the lesion persists, enlarges, or causes pain is it necessary to carry out an excision biopsy, usually under local anaesthesia.

Accessory nipples

The breast develops from the milk line which extends from axilla to inguinal region. Usually there is degeneration of the mammary cells other than on the anterior chest wall, but islands of cells may form accessory breast tissue. The commonest site for accessory breast tissue is the axilla, with or without an

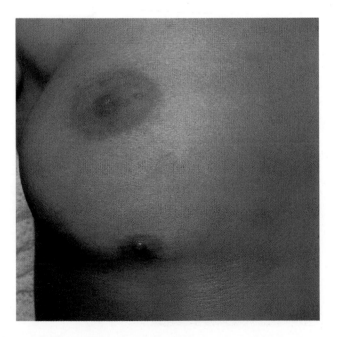

Figure 2.2

A well-developed nipple–areolar complex.

accessory nipple. The next most common site is inframammary and this is the usual site for a rudimentary nipple, and occasionally a well-developed nipple–areolar complex. Only rarely are these found in the inguinal region, the most famous bearer of an inguinal nipple being Anne Boleyn.

Unilateral inversion

Confronted with a patient complaining of recent onset of unilateral nipple inversion, it should be checked whether it is possible to evert the nipple. If this is possible, it is unlikely that there is serious underlying pathology. Additionally, the aim of examination is to determine whether there is an associated mass.

Sometimes the inverted nipple may itself give the impression of a mass. If there is a mass and nipple inversion this is a grave sign and suggests underlying cancer. In postmenopausal women with transverse indrawing of the nipple and no mass, the likely diagnosis is duct ectasia. The presence of a nipple discharge should be sought and, if present, tested for the presence of

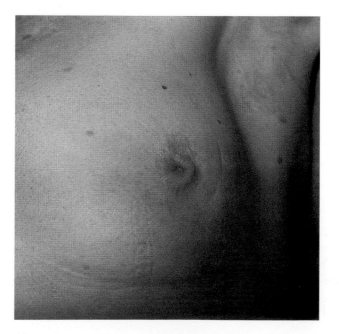

Figure 2.3

A case of unilateral nipple inversion. Note the whitish substance which is due to retention of skin secretion.

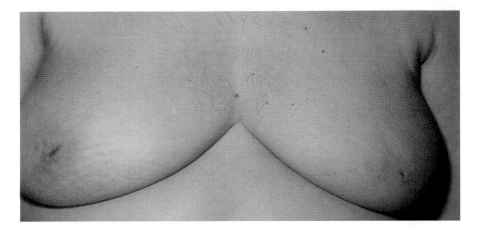

Figure 2.4

Bilateral nipple inversion.

occult blood. Nipple inversion is commonly associated with a crusting smelly discharge due to retention of skin secretions.

Bilateral inversion

Probably the commonest cause of bilateral nipple inversion is idiopathic, with the patient giving a history of inversion since puberty and being unable to breast feed her children. Later onset of bilateral nipple inversion is due to duct ectasia. Cancer is almost never a cause of bilateral nipple inversion.

Paget's disease of nipple

This is classically a scaly, itchy eczematous reaction on the nipple, not associated with eczema elsewhere. With progression the disease also involves the areola. The nipple may be raw and sometimes inverted. The diagnosis is confirmed by wedge biopsy under local anaesthesia. If Paget's disease is associated with a mass, it is usually due to invasive carcinoma. When there is Paget's with no associated lump there is underlying ductal

11

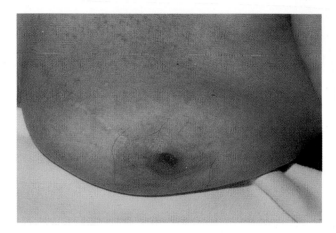

Figure 2.5

A case of Paget's disease of the nipple with no areolar involvement.

carcinoma in situ (DCIS) in approximately 50% of cases and invasive cancer in the remainder.

The usual treatment is a modified radical mastectomy since there may be

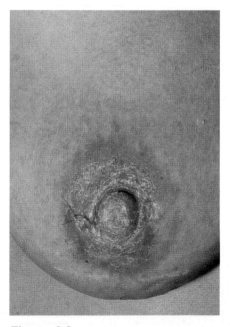

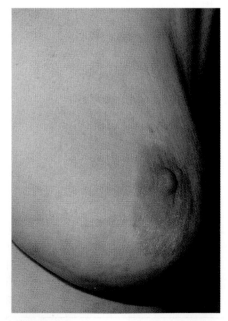

Figure 2.6

A case of extensive Paget's disease of the nipple–areolar complex.

Figure 2.7

A case of eczema of the areola. Note the nipple-sparing phenomena in benign eczema of the breast.

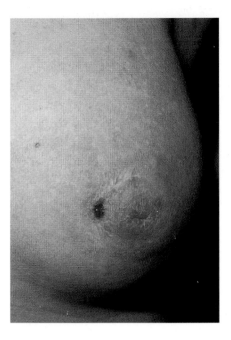

Figure 2.8

A case of mammary fistula in a 26-year-old woman. The patient is a smoker and the fistula was established after recurrent para-areolar sepsis treated by antibiotics.

multicentric disease and axillary nodal involvement is a frequent event when the underlying disease is invasive. Paget's is the result of migration of malignant cells beneath the basement membrane onto the skin surface. Pathologically they are recognised as large cells with ballooned nuclei. Eczematous changes of the areola sparing the nipple are rarely the result of Paget's disease.

Mammillary fistula

This often unrecognised disease can give rise to substantial morbidity, with patients undergoing repeated drainage of abscesses and resection of breast tissue. When correctly diagnosed and treated, the patient can be cured. Typically the patient is in her twenties or thirties, is a smoker, and may or may not have had a yellow nipple discharge. A breast abscess develops, and surgical incision and drainage is performed. The wound may appear to heal, but within a few weeks another periareolar abscess occurs. Successive attempts at drainage with or without antibiotics do not achieve long-term cure.

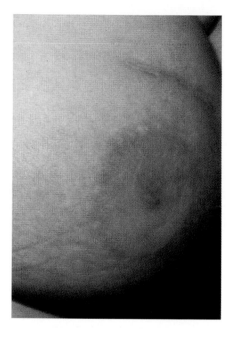

Figure 2.9
Depigmentation following radiotherapy to the left breast. Note the tumorectomy scar.

The problem is that a blind-ending sac of infection persists deep to the areola which discharges through the fistulous opening at the areolar margin. To enable the mammillary fistula to heal, a probe has to be inserted from the

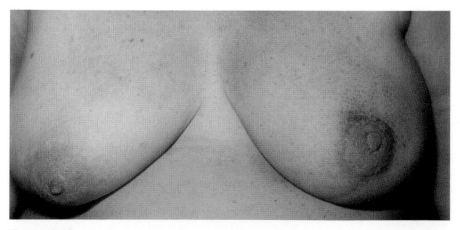

Figure 2.10
Radiotherapy to the breast may also lead to hyperpigmentation, as seen in this case.

para-areolar sinus through to the nipple and the tract laid open and its base excised and edges trimmed (saucerisation of fistula). The cavity is packed regularly and allowed to granulate from the base. Once this has occurred the mammillary fistula almost never recurs. An alternative approach is to excise the fistulous tract followed by primary closure under antibiotic cover.

Nipple depigmentation

The usual reason for depigmentation of the nipple is external irradiation as part of breast conservation therapy (BCT). Whereas there may be darkening of irradiated skin in some cases, there is a loss of pigment from the nipple–areolar complex. A rarer cause is vitiligo specifically affecting the nipple. Usually no treatment is required other than reassurance, but in selected unilateral cases tattooing may be considered.

KEY POINTS

- Recent unilateral nipple inversion needs special evaluation.
- Eczema, crusting or bleeding may be due to Paget's disease.
- Recurrent periareolar abscesses arise from a mammillary fistula.

3
NIPPLE DISCHARGE

Algorithm of management

In patients who complain of a nipple discharge it is important to enquire about its colour, whether it is unilateral or bilateral, and whether it was found because of staining on the bra, or has been noted whilst bathing, spontaneous, or non-spontaneous. This gives some indication of the volume of discharge. If there is a palpable breast lump this needs to be investigated. In the absence of any masses the laterality of the discharge should be noted, together with its emergence from a single or multiple ducts.

Irrespective of colour, the discharge, unless frankly blood stained, should be tested for the presence of haemoglobin. This is carried out with a urine

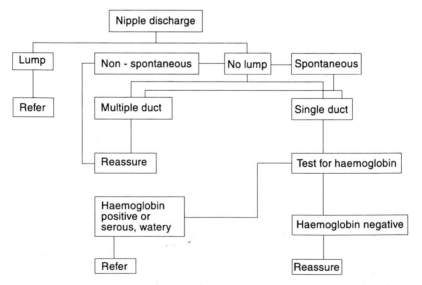

Figure 3.1

Management of nipple discharge.

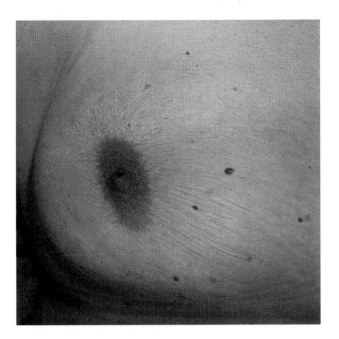

Figure 3.2
A case of frank bloody nipple discharge.

testing stick. Special attention should be paid to serous or watery discharges, since these are more likely to be associated with an underlying malignancy. If the discharge is from multiple ducts, or is haemoglobin negative and derived from a single duct, the patient can be reassured.

Should the discharge prove to contain haemoglobin, surgical intervention is indicated. The isolated duct and lobule are excised, through a circumareolar incision (microdochectomy). This serves to relieve the patient of the discharge and also provides a histological diagnosis.

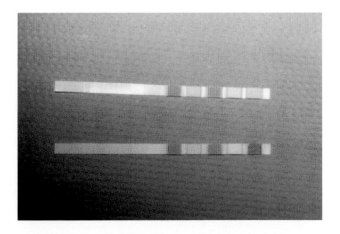

Figure 3.3
Urine testing stick showing change of colour to green in cases of discharge with occult blood.

In patients with a blood-containing discharge without a palpable lump, one-third will have an intraduct papilloma, one-third duct ectasia, and one-third fibrocystic disease. Only 5% will have cancers, half of these being ductal carcinomas in situ and the rest invasive.

Normal lactation

Not surprisingly the commonest cause of nipple discharge is physiological, namely lactation. Occasionally, when lactation starts there is some blood staining. Almost always this is not serious and settles spontaneously. It is not necessary for the woman to stop breast feeding. This may occur also during pregnancy and occasionally in women taking the oral contraceptive pill.

Involution of lactating breast tissue is variable once breast feeding ceases. Many women continue to have a small amount of milky discharge for many months, sometimes years, after lactating. No treatment is required and they can be reassured that their discharge is physiological.

Galactorrhoea

Physiological milky discharge becomes pathological when it is so profuse that the patient has to wear pads in her bra all the time and when there is associated menstrual irregularity. This combination is suspicious of hyperprolactinaemia as a result of a pituitary adenoma.

A timed blood sample is sent for prolactin estimation (there is diurnal variation). If this shows an elevation of prolactin the pituitary fossa is X-rayed to exclude a large adenoma. More frequently there is a microadenoma, detectable on CT or MRI scan. First-line treatment is medical using bromocriptine or one of the new D2 dopamine agonists, which results in normalisation of the prolactin level and resolution of the galactorrhoea. Surgery or radiotherapy are rarely necessary.

Yellow discharge

This is typically seen in patients with duct ectasia, or its variant periductal mastitis in younger women complaining of a yellow-coloured discharge, and

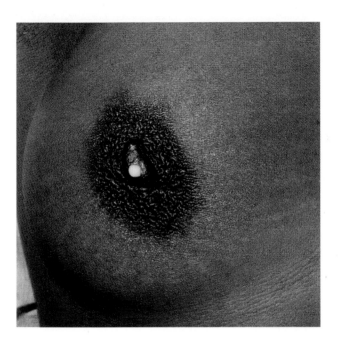

Figure 3.4
Galactorrhoea.

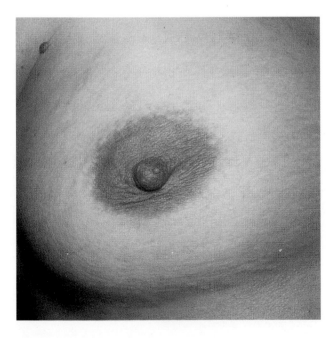

Figure 3.5
A case of yellow
discharge.

frequently arises from multiple ducts. This may be associated with breast discomfort and sometimes with unilateral nipple inversion. Provided that there are no palpable masses, the discharge is haemoglobin negative and mammograms are normal, the patient can be reassured. Patients with duct ectasia should be urged to stop smoking, since this affects the bacterial flora and puts them at increased risk of breast abscess and subsequent mammillary fistula.

Yellow discharge may be mistakenly thought to be purulent. In the absence of signs of acute inflammmation, antibiotics are not required since they do not have any impact on the volume or colour of the discharge. This type of discharge does not originate from infection; it is the more concentrated form of physiological discharge which has been lying stagnant in dilated ducts.

Clear discharge

Discharge of a clear, straw-coloured nature is almost invariably associated with occult blood positivity. The usual cause of such a discharge is an intraduct papilloma and this is both diagnosed and treated by

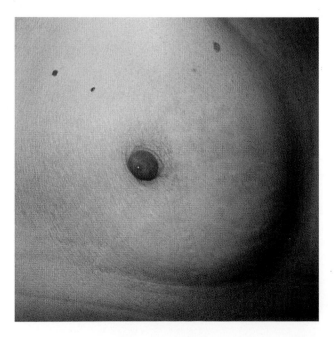

Figure 3.6

A case of clear discharge. Examination revealed no other abnormality. This proved to be a case of intraductal papilloma.

microdochectomy. Single intraduct papillomas are not a risk factor for breast cancer and patients do not need close follow up. In contrast, multiple papillomatosis is a premalignant condition, and such patients should remain under surveillance.

A straw-coloured discharge released from a palpable mass, is a serious sign, usually indicative that there is an intraduct carcinoma (ductal carcinoma in situ) or an invasive cancer. Such patients need urgent referral to a breast clinic.

KEY POINTS

- The commonest cause of bilateral nipple discharge is lactation or incomplete involution afterwards.
- Patients with a blood-containing discharge from a single duct require referral, irrespective of the colour of the discharge.

4
BREAST PAIN

The commonest breast symptom for which women consult their GPs is breast pain, usually of a cyclical nature. Most often in premenopausal women this is a more extreme variant of premenstrual discomfort and lasts for a short time before resolving spontaneously. A similar situation can occur in postmenopausal women taking hormone replacement therapy (HRT).

In postmenopausal women not taking HRT the commonest causes of mastalgia are duct ectasia and referred pain from the underlying rib cage. While it is normally assumed that if the patient has a lump or lumpiness with associated pain that this will not be malignant, it should be remembered that one in ten patients with breast cancer will complain of some discomfort, usually a localised burning sensation.

Various classifications of mastalgia, of varying complexity, have been suggested. Probably the simplest is separation into three groups: cyclical, non-cyclical, and extramammary. Usually the patient will be able to state whether the pain is cyclical in nature, but sometimes it is necessary to ask them to keep a breast pain and menstrual calendar.

Clinical examination may be completely normal, or there may be an associated area of tender nodularity. There is no relationship between the apparent extent of nodularity and the severity of the pain. Just because the patient complains of severe pain, yet has no apparent clinical signs does not mean that the pain is hysterical in nature.

If no lumps are present, or there is slight nodularity, the patient can be reassured by the general practitioner and reviewed 6 weeks later, by which time many will have improved or be pain free. Should there be a more definite area of tender nodularity the patient should be seen in 3 weeks. Those in whom the nodularity is more pronounced should be referred to a breast clinic for evaluation.

Algorithm of management

For the majority of women with mastalgia the management will comprise history taking, examination, and sympathetic reassurance. The omission of any of these vital steps will lead to increased patient anxiety with frequent return for consultation and an increased number of unnecessary hospital referrals.

Only a few of these patients require specific therapy. Once they have been reassured that their pain is not due to serious underlying pathology and they are not at increased risk of subsequent breast cancer, most will not want any treatment.

Similarly, postmenopausal patients with breast pain referred from the rib cage are usually reassured to learn that their breasts are normal. Such an occasion provides an opportunity for the doctor to encourage the patient to take part in the National Breast Cancer Screening Programme.

The few women who do need treatment are those who have self-rated moderate or severe breast pain which has persisted for 6 months or more.

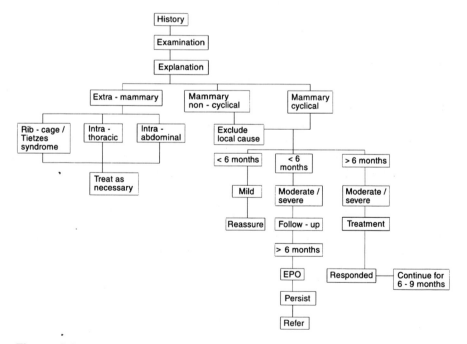

Figure 4.1.

Management of mastalgia. EPO = evening primrose oil

The pain will trouble them to the extent that they cannot let their partner touch them, are unable to hug their children, and may avoid public transport because of fear of being jostled.

Sometimes, as the doctor approaches at the start of the breast examination, the patient will involuntarily cross her arms on the chest because of fear of being touched. When this sign is elicited, intervention is needed. For such a case, successful treatment can change her life.

Site of pain

The patient is asked to indicate the location of the pain. Commonly those with chronic mastalgia have bilateral pain, but it is unilateral in 40% of cases. Often the pain radiates through to the nipples and down the arms. When the pain is localised it should be established whether it is within or deep to the breast tissue. Sometimes as the examiner's finger is placed on the site this induces more pain (trigger point). Again, it should be determined whether this point lies within the breast or underneath, by lifting the breast tissue away from the underlying rib cage. This may be easier to achieve by examining the patient in the lateral position.

Exclusion of extramammary pathology

Many extramammary lesions give rise to breast pain. The commonest is musculoskeletal disease and this is usually apparent after a careful clinical examination. Less commonly, angina, gall stones, and hiatus hernia can be responsible, and the pain may be worse after exercise or in relation to the ingestion of food. Another exacerbating factor is endogenous depression when the patient has an enhanced awareness of normal cyclical changes.

Tietze's syndrome

This condition is the result of osteochondritis at the costo-chondral junction and may give rise to unilateral or bilateral pain on the medial aspect of the breast. On palpation, there is localised tenderness over one or more costo-chondral junctions, and gentle pressure reproduces the pain of which the patient complains. Usually the pain is self-limiting but sometimes, if protracted, it may help to give a local injection of both steroid and local anaesthetic.

Radiculitis

Localised, laterally located pain, sometimes radiating around the chest wall, may arise from an intercostal nerve, trapped between rib and intercostal muscle. The site of pain may be very limited and the pain may be exacerbated by asking the patient to elevate her arm. Treatment is usually by reassurance but a few patients may benefit from a local injection. Such pain may occur after chronic chest infection and some patients will give a history of prior rib trauma.

Therapies

The majority of women with pain of mammary origin will require reassurance and no specific therapy. If the mastalgia persists for 6 months or more, there may be benefit in giving treatment. Non-effective therapies include antibiotics, diuretics, vitamin B6, and vitamin E.

Treatment should be started with an effective but non-toxic therapy, namely, evening primrose oil (EPO). This relieves symptoms in approximately 50% of women with mild/moderate pain. The patient should be warned that benefit may not be apparent immediately. A minimum of 3 months' treatment should be given at a dosage of 240 mg/day of gamolenic acid, before deciding that EPO will not work.

For patients with mastalgia which is refractory to EPO, treatment options include danazol, bromocriptine, and tamoxifen. The former two agents are licensed for this indication but can give rise to side effects in a substantial proportion of cases. The key to minimising side effects is to start at the lowest possible dose and only increase if this does not work. The recommended dose of danazol is 100 mg daily, which can subsequently be reduced to every other day. Gradual administration of bromocriptine starting with 1·25 mg daily, doubled every 4 days to a maximum of 5 mg daily, will reduce the severity of side effects.

Tamoxifen is not licensed for mastalgia, but at a dosage of 10 mg daily it relieves mastalgia very quickly with very few side effects. Once patients understand that the agent works for them the dose can be reduced to 10 mg on alternate days, and in some cases the drug is taken only when the patient is aware that the pain is imminent. Since tamoxifen induces ovulation patients must use a barrier form of contraception. Oral contraceptives can be taken safely with EPO but not with any other antimastalgia drugs.

The GnRH analogue goserelin relieves refractory breast pain in the majority of cases but is associated with severe menopausal symptoms and measurable bone loss. Studies are underway to examine 'add-back', whereby a combination of goserelin and oestrogen is given. This approach remains experimental.

KEY POINTS

- Most patients with cyclical mastalgia need reassurance not therapy.
- Most older patients with breast pain have a musculoskeletal cause.
- If symptoms are moderate or severe and have been present for 6 months or more, try evening primrose oil.
- For refractory pain use danazol or bromocriptine, or refer to a specialised clinic.

5
BREAST LUMPS IN YOUNG WOMEN

There will be differing views on what constitutes a young woman. In the context of breast disease, this will be taken as those aged up to 35 years of age. The reasons for this are that mammography is agreed to be of little use in evaluation for this age group, and also such women carry a higher risk of recurrence after breast conservation treatment for malignancy, and finally are more likely to have poorly differentiated cancers with a bad prognosis.

Luckily, cancer is rare in this age group, but it is important that young women with discrete lumps or localised nodularity are not dismissed as having a fibroadenoma or fibroadenosis without appropriate investigations being carried out.

History taking

The commonest complaint in this age group will be breast tenderness with or without associated lumpiness. Some will complain of a painless lump and, particularly in those under 25 years, it is likely to be a fibroadenoma.

Breast cysts are unusual in these women other than galactocoeles in lactating women. Very painful lumps are rare, except for the few who develop an acute abscess, usually when lactating but sometimes as a consequence of nipple inversion and periductal mastitis.

An important condition to be aware of is unilateral subareolar swelling in a prepubertal girl. This is the result of asynchronous growth of the breast bud. Reassurance is required. Anyone foolish enough to excise such a lump will be responsible for unilateral non-development of the breast.

Fibroadenoma

This classic breast lump of postpubertal females is the result of overgrowth of a lobule. Normally it is painless and freely mobile, moving away from the examiner's fingers, hence its nickname 'breast mouse'. The texture is smooth but often lobulated, with well-defined margins. Once a fibroadenoma is greater than 1 cm diameter its nature is usually apparent. Smaller lesions which appear smooth and apparently mobile will sometimes prove to be poorly differentiated (ductal grade III) cancers.

Although the diagnosis can be made clinically, confirmation of this is required if the lump is not going to be removed. Obviously many young women will wish to avoid surgery, providing that they can be reassured that the lump is benign and does not place them at increased risk of subsequent malignancy. This means that it is essential that malignant lesions masquerading in benign guise are identified.

The nature of a smooth mobile breast lump should be confirmed by both ultrasound and fine needle aspiration cytology. Then the patient can be told that surgery is unnecessary provided that the lump does not increase in size or become painful. Despite this reassurance, follow-up studies have shown that, eventually, approximately 50% of women with a clinical fibroadenoma will have the lump removed.

Giant fibroadenoma

A giant fibroadenoma is described as a lobulated mobile lesion, greater than 3 cm diameter, and showing rapid increase in size, often with associated pain. Normally they occur in adolescents and can be a cause of great concern to the patient and her mother. Treatment is by surgery and, provided that excision has been complete, recurrence is rare.

A source of confusion is the phyllodes tumour, once known as cystosarcoma phylloides. These lumps which usually occur in older women may appear as fibroadenomas, and may seem to enucleate at the time of surgery. Unfortunately, tongues of tissue are left behind and recurrence is invariable. Wide excision is necessary, and sometimes a total mastectomy. Local behaviour of phyllodes tumours does not correlate well with the histological appearance.

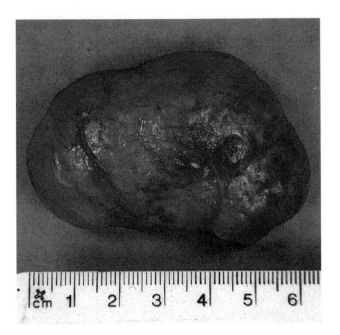

Figure 5.1
Giant fibroadenoma.

Lumps during lactation

Usually lumps which occur during lactation are areas of benign nodularity. Nevetheless, evaluation of the lactating breast can be difficult and such cases should be referred for specialist evaluation. Sometimes pre-existing fibroadenomas will undergo a growth spurt during lactation and may mimic a cancer. Cancers are rare, so the examiner's index of suspicion is low. If there is any doubt an expert opinion should be sought.

The sudden development of a discrete lump in a lactating woman is usually a milk cyst, galactocoele. If this is suspected a needle is inserted and if milk, sometimes inspissated, is drained and the lump disappears, the condition has been both diagnosed and also treated.

However, a note of warning should be sounded. It is important that the attempted drainage of the putative milk cyst is carried out by the person who will be responsible for excising the lesion, should it prove to be solid. Aspiration of a lactating breast may give rise to bleeding and the resulting haematoma may alter the clinical signs, turning what might be an operable carcinoma into an inoperable lesion. Caveat aspirator.

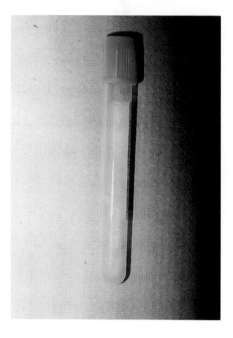

Figure 5.2

Milky fluid aspirated from a galactocele with total disappearance of the mass.

Carcinoma

Young women with breast cancer suffer from two disadvantages. Firstly, their disease may often be diagnosed after some delay because nobody considered that they might have breast cancer. Secondly, they are more likely to have an aggressive breast cancer. For these reasons a disproportionate number die of breast cancer.

Thus a balance must be reached between needlessly worrying the majority of young women and mistakenly reassuring those with malignancy. Women with discrete lumps need hospital evaluation, irrespective of age. More problematical are those with nodularity. It is important that if there is any doubt in the examiner's mind the patient is brought back for review within 3 weeks so that a second examination is carried out.

If a decision is made to operate on a suspicious lump in a young woman, it is better that an excision biopsy, rather than core needle biopsy, be carried out. If possible, the examination should be carried out in the luteal phase of the menstrual cycle.

KEY POINTS

- The commonest lump in young women is a fibroadenoma.
- Fibroadenomas can be treated conservatively, provided that they are clinically, cytologically and ultrasonically benign.
- Patients with localised persistent nodularity need specialised evaluation.
- Pregnant women with breast lumps need urgent evaluation.

6
BREAST LUMPS IN MIDDLE-AGED WOMEN

Middle age is difficult to define. If women between 35 and 55 are taken to be middle aged, most are aware that breast cancer is the commonest cause of death among their peer group. Thus breast symptoms may be very alarming for such women, as many will have friends or relatives who have died from the disease. As an additional complication, most will be premenopausal or taking hormone replacement therapy so that cyclical changes may be present.

Almost any form of breast pathology can occur in this group. The commonest cause of breast lumps is localised nodularity, which is often part of a more generalised process. Sudden-onset painful lumps are usually cysts. Non-painful smooth lumps may prove to be fibroadenomas, but these can be mimicked by cancers. Even small but discrete lumps cannot be ignored in this age group unless they have been shown unequivocally to be benign.

Irrespective of the clinical findings, most centres offer bilateral mammography to women over 40, although some have ceased ordering this investigation in women under 50 since no reduction in mortality has been shown after screening women in this age group.

History taking

The time and manner of discovery of the lump should be sought, together with its relationship to the menstrual cycle. It should be determined whether the lump has increased in size since presentation, there is associated nipple discharge/inversion, and there is change in shape of the breast. Prior breast surgery should be noted and the family history sought, in particular the age at diagnosis of first-degree relatives, when known. Additionally, it is important to ask about present or recent use of oral contraceptives or hormone replacement therapy.

Localised nodularity

This condition is the commonest cause of breast lumps in this age group. It is also known as fibroadenosis and is a region of thickening without an edge, although sometimes it may appear to be discrete when located on the periphery of the breast. Often there is localised tenderness which may be cyclical and associated with increased swelling premenstrually. Tissue deficit at the site of a previous biopsy may also give the impression of a lump with an edge.

Provided that fine needle aspiration cytology (FNAC) shows benign epithelial cells and mammograms are normal, the patient can be reassured. Should the FNAC specimen be inadequate, or the mammograms equivocal, it may be necessary to carry out an excision biopsy. A Trucut biopsy is not a good method of proving the benign nature of a lump, because of sampling limitations. Indeed a benign Trucut biopsy from an equivocal lump is an indication for open biopsy.

Fibroadenoma

Although these lumps usually present at a younger age, some previously undetected fibroadenomas will be found in well woman clinics or on screening mammograms. In middle-aged women they are usually removed, but if there is ultrasonic and cytological evidence confirming their benign

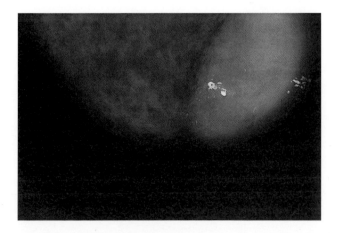

Figure 6.1

Benign macro-calcification in a large fibroadenoma.

nature, surgery can be avoided. If the mammogram shows macrocalcification within a well-defined opacity, this is diagnostic of fibroadenoma.

Cyst

A substantial number of women have breast cysts which are asymptomatic and are picked up by ultrasound or suspected on mammography. Typically women with symptomatic cysts are aged over 35, still menstruating, or taking HRT. Many will state that they suddenly became aware of a breast lump, because of sudden onset of localised tenderness.

Although the lump may be smooth and mobile, it can also appear somewhat irregular, particularly in women with nodular breasts. Cystic disease is likely when there is more than one lump or if the patient gives a prior history of gross cysts. However, it is important to be aware that women with multiple cysts are at increased risk of breast cancer. Thus these lumps do need evaluation.

Treatment is simple. A needle is inserted into the cyst and aspiration performed. If cyst fluid is obtained and the lump disappears, both diagnosis

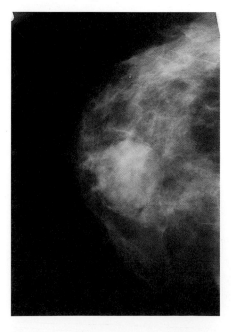

Figure 6.2

Mammographic appearance of a cyst. Note the well-defined margins. The diagnosis was confirmed by successful aspiration.

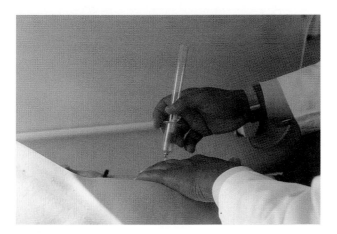

Figure 6.3
A cyst being
evaluated using the
vacutainer system.

and treatment have been achieved. Cyst fluid can be of various colours, yellow, green, or brown. Provided that there is no blood in the cyst fluid and that the lump is impalpable after aspiration, it is not necessary to send the fluid for cytology. Cystic carcinomas contain blood and do not disappear.

The patient is reviewed 6 weeks later and provided that there is no recurrence of the lump, she can be reassured. However, if the same cyst

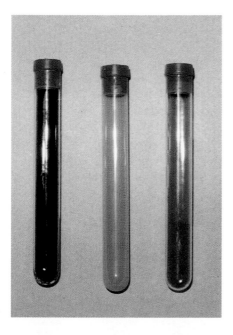

Figure 6.4
Cyst fluid.

recurs more than once, excision biopsy should be arranged. Mammograms can be useful in determining the presence of other cysts so that the patient can be warned that she may develop subsequent cysts and in this event will require re-evaluation. Occasionally, there may be a concomitant impalpable carcinoma.

Should GPs aspirate breast cysts? It would seem very reasonable and a great saving of time and worry for the patient, if the GP was to aspirate the suspected cyst in the surgery using a syringe and needle. However, there is a problem. If the suspected cyst is solid, the act of aspiration may cause a haematoma and this may change the size of the lump and occasionally produce skin change.

Thus if the lump proves eventually to be a carcinoma it may be iatrogenically up-staged and a patient may have an unnecessary mastectomy or redundant first-line chemotherapy. The person aspirating the cyst should also be responsible for carrying out further treatment should the lump be solid. An alteration in the clinical signs following a well-meant attempt to aspirate may not be in the patient's long-term interests.

Carcinoma

Although it is taught that breast cancers are painless lumps, one in ten will be painful, usually of a burning nature, and some will not be discrete hard irregular lumps. Infiltrating lobular carcinoma can be difficult to diagnose. The cells infiltrate diffusely in an Indian-file manner and may not elicit a fibrous reaction, so that the lump is not hard and may be poorly defined. Additionally, the cancer may not be apparent on a mammogram, and because the cells are in single file, they may be difficult to obtain on FNAC.

However the majority of cancers in this age group will be non-tender lumps and some may be difficult to distinguish from cysts, hence the advice in the previous section. If there is clinical evidence of infiltration such as skin tethering, deep fixation, nipple retraction, or enlarged/fixed axillary nodes, the patient can be told the likely diagnosis at that time. FNAC, or core needle biopsy, can then be used to make the diagnosis, after which treatment options can be discussed.

For the majority of patients there will not be any definite evidence of invasion, and so FNAC alone will not be sufficient to determine the nature of the cancer in terms of whether it is in situ or invasive. Thus a histological diagnosis should be made. Work from Guy's Hospital suggests that if a histological diagnosis is to be made in a premenopausal woman, it should be carried out in the luteal phase of the menstrual cycle. As a counsel of perfection, it may be best that any invasive procedures are carried out in the latter half of the cycle in patients other than those with irregular periods or who are taking the pill or HRT.

After an excision biopsy has been performed the specimen should be processed for paraffin section and not frozen section. There is no need to proceed immediately to a definitive procedure in women with early breast cancer. Frozen section is a suboptimal method of fixation and may pressurise the pathologist into making a diagnosis on an inadequately prepared slide.

The delay means that the patient has more time to come to terms with the likely diagnosis and treatment options can be discussed fully, with time for support from a nurse counsellor. There is no evidence that a delay of up to 4 weeks before biopsy and definitive treatment has any prejudicial effect on prognosis.

KEY POINTS

- Middle-aged women with breast lumps need urgent referral.
- Persistent localised nodularity should be evaluated in a breast clinic.
- Women starting HRT do not need referral to a breast clinic.
- Suspected breast cysts should not be aspirated routinely by GPs.

7
BREAST LUMPS IN OLDER WOMEN

Breast lumps in older women have to be regarded as malignant until proven otherwise. However, who are the elderly? In terms of clinical research, older women have been defined as those over 70, since they have been excluded from the majority of prospective randomised trials. From the screening point of view, those over 65 are elderly and cease to be in the call-recall system.

There are many misconceptions concerning the nature of breast cancer in the elderly. Many regard the disease as being more indolent 'atrophic scirrhous cancer', and assume that the patient will live out her natural lifespan without problems from the carcinoma. Unfortunately, this is not true. Some elderly patients have slow-growing breast cancers, but most have cancers that can be as equally lethal as those in their younger sisters.

Others regard aggressive treatment as being an inappropriate option for the elderly because of co-morbidity increasing the risk of either surgery or radiotherapy. Again, this stereotype is unhelpful. The majority of older women are fit enough for a general anaesthetic to enable extensive surgery, if necessary. Radiotherapy is an intrinsic part of breast conservation therapy but is often withheld in the elderly because of fears of excess morbidity and the possible need for hospitalisation, thereby blocking a bed. There is no evidence to support this.

Paradoxically, others assume that if a mastectomy is suggested this will not cause psychological problems in older women, because they will not be concerned about breast conservation. This assumption is also fallacious, with many older patients being very keen to preserve their body image.

To overcome some of these problems, the agent tamoxifen has been used extensively, in order to avoid or minimise surgery and radiotherapy, since the majority of older patients will have hormone-sensitive tumours. The hope was that the tamoxifen would maintain the disease in remission either permanently or for long enough that death from other causes would intervene.

It was also assumed that a subsequent salvage mastectomy would be possible and that progression or relapse of disease would not have any impact on prognosis. Clinical trials have shown that these assumptions were not at all justified.

History taking

Although some elderly patients will find the breast lump themselves, many of them are detected by their GP as part of a routine clinical examination when the patient complains of, say, a chest infection. It should be remembered that approximately 40% of all breast cancer cases are aged over 70 at the time of diagnosis. Thus this is an age group that is worth checking for the presence of breast lumps.

Breast examination is made more easy by the fatty replacement that occurs as the breast undergoes postmenopausal involution. However, this may also lead to the emergence of benign lesions such as fibroadenomas, which have been previously cocooned in normal breast tissue.

Apart from lumps, many elderly patients will complain of breast pain. In this age group, extramammary causes such as angina or arthritis are likely to be responsible, but it is important that the breasts are examined to exclude a palpable lump.

Unilateral nipple inversion may be a worrying symptom for the patient. With or without a palpable lump they should be referred for evaluation. Eventually some will be diagnosed with duct ectasia for which no treatment will be required but many will prove to have underlying malignancy.

Benign breast cysts are rare in elderly women but the incidence is increasing due to the use of HRT. Large blue cysts containing blood may be the presenting feature of papillary carcinoma, which is more common in elderly patients.

Localised nodularity

In this age group there may be involution at a slower rate in one breast so that it is more nodular, usually in the upper outer quadrant. Although benign, such cases require evaluation, usually by examination and mammography and sometimes FNAC. Such nodularity may be more marked and associated with tenderness in those taking HRT.

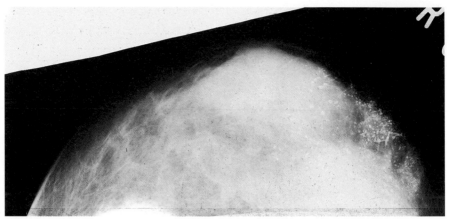

Figure 7.1
A typical appearance of malignant calcification. Note the irregularity in shape and density.

Mammography

Fatty replacement of breast tissue helps both clinical and radiological investigation of breasts in the elderly. Additionally, at a subjective level the compression involved in mammography will cause less discomfort. X-rays may demonstrate unsuspected involuting and calcifying fibroadenomas. This appearance is typical and no further investigation is required.

More serious is the detection of microcalcification with or without an associated mass. When this is found the patient should be re-examined, since such a lesion may be palpable once the examiner's attention has been drawn to the appropriate quadrant.

At present, detection of asymptomatic ductal carcinoma in situ in older women is unusual. This may be because the condition is less frequent with increasing age, but may reflect the decreased use of mammography in this age group.

Core needle biopsy

A variety of devices is available for taking a tissue core. The original was Trucut, which is still used extensively. It has a sensitivity of 80% and a specificity of 100%. However, because of the need to fix the tumour and also

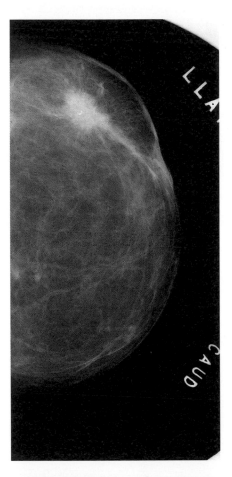

Figure 7.2
A typical appearance of breast cancer. Note the irregular outline as well as drawn-in nipple.

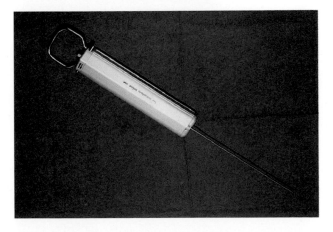

Figure 7.3
The Bioptycut system ready to use.

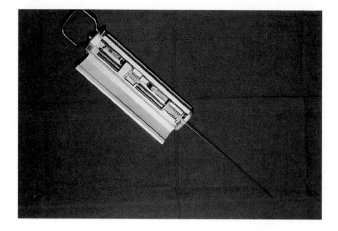

Figure 7.4

The Bioptycut system
with the lid open and
the needle mounted.

move the outer cutting sheath, there is a risk of crush artefact which can
render histological interpretation impossible.

The Bioptycut system overcomes this problem by being spring-loaded.
Core needle biopsy can be used not only to make a histological diagnosis
before conservation therapy or mastectomy, but also in patients with larger
tumours who may be candidates for first-line chemotherapy. Additionally,
oestrogen and progesterone receptor status can be measured on the
specimens, so that appropriate subsequent therapy can be planned.

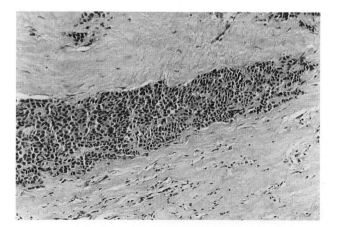

Figure 7.5

A tissue core showing
breast cancer.

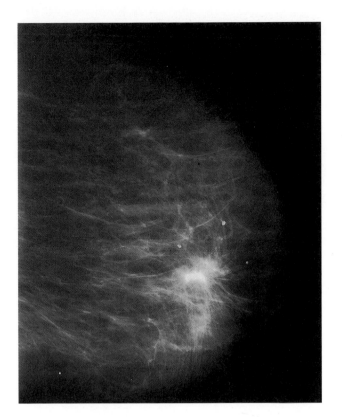

Figure 7.6

A mammogram of fat necrosis mimicking carcinoma following breast cancer therapy.

Fine needle aspiration cytology (FNAC)

This procedure is used in most centres to make a diagnosis of malignancy. It is a very useful diagnostic test, but results need to be applied with thought if inappropriate treatments are to be avoided. If clinical evidence of invasion is present and cytology is positive, definitive treatment can be discussed. When FNAC is positive but the clinical signs are of a lump or area of nodularity, histology is required to make the full diagnosis. Treatment should not be instigated without this.

Particularly problematical are women who have had breast conservation treatment and are suspected to have local relapse. Clinical signs may suggest a lump, radiology may show a mass with associated distortion, and cytology may be atypical. This is insufficient evidence to allow salvage mastectomy to be performed. Under these circumstances a frozen section is required before mastectomy is carried out.

The technique of FNAC appears deceptively simple, but substantial improvements in adequacy of samples occurs with experience. Wet-fixed smears are stained with Papanicolaou stain, and air-dried specimens with May–Grünwald–Giemsa.

KEY POINTS

- Elderly women with breast lumps have cancer until proven otherwise.
- A lump arising after trauma may be a haematoma but malignancy must be excluded.
- Longstanding nipple inversion is not in itself an indication for referral to a breast clinic.

8
SKIN

Erythema

Redness of the skin is one of the four cardinal signs of acute inflammation. Thus when skin erythema develops over the breast it may be an indicator of an acute abscess. Other than in lactating women, such infections are rare but may occur in smokers with periductal mastitis or older women with duct ectasia. When accompanied by a tender lump, and sometimes painful axillary lymphadenopathy, the diagnosis may be made by aspirating pus from the lump. This may obviate the need for incision and drainage. Such abscesses are usually of staphylococcal aetiology and respond to treatment with flucloxacillin.

Erythema may occur in florid fibroadenosis when there is a sudden painful swelling of the breast which is hormonal in origin but which resolves spontaneously. Antibiotics are not necessary. An erysipeloid reaction may occur sometimes in patients with carcinoma, and usually a less florid reaction is associated with skin oedema in inflammatory carcinoma. It is usual for skin erythema to occur in the radiation field of patients undergoing breast conservation therapy.

Peau d'orange

Skin oedema (*peau d'orange*) is the result of obstruction to the lymphatic drainage of the skin which gives rise to the characteristic appearance. When associated with a breast lump it is highly suggestive of malignancy. If directly overlying the lump and localised, the disease may still be operable. If *peau d'orange* is more extensive than the lump, or is at a distance from it, usually inferior, the disease is inoperable. Good light is necessary to elicit this clinical sign. *Peau d'orange* can develop after a needle biopsy so that it is particularly

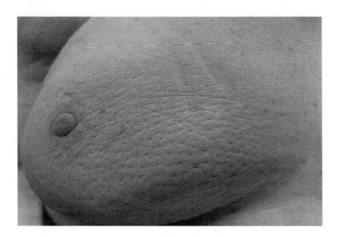

Figure 8.1

Erythema and *peau d'orange* as a manifestation of locally advanced breast cancer.

important that clinical signs are recorded accurately at the time of first presentation so that the patient is not subsequently staged wrongly.

Mock orange

There may be an appearance of the skin over the sternum which mimics *peau d'orange* and has been dubbed mock orange syndrome (*Philadelphus* sp.).

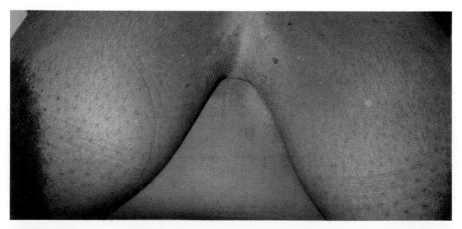

Figure 8.2

A case of mock orange syndrome. Note the breast size, bilaterality and medial location.

46

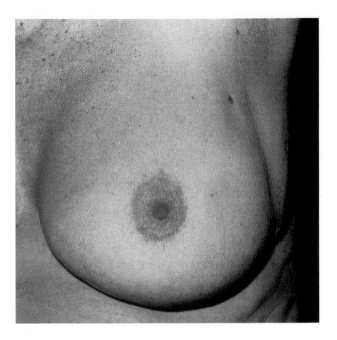

Figure 8.3
Skin dimpling seen
only on elevation of
the arm.

This is a frequent finding in women with and without breast lumps and needs
to be remembered as an innocent artefact.

Skin tethering

One of the signs that women are told to look for when examining their breasts
is any skin puckering or distortion. When skin tethering is seen in association
with a lump, this is very suspicious of cancer, although it may occur with an
acute abscess, or where there has been previous surgery. Occasionally there
may be a suspicion of skin tethering associated with fat necrosis following
trauma to the breast.

Mondor's syndrome

Skin tethering may not be associated with any palpable lump and may result
from localised thrombophlebitis of a lateral thoracic vein. There may be some

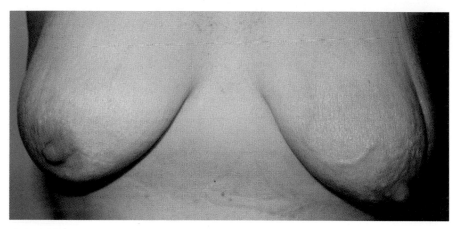

Figure 8.4
A case of Mondor's syndrome. Note the characteristic longitudinal dimpling.

prior tenderness and sometimes slight discolouration around a linear puckering usually on the lateral aspect of the breast. The patient does not normally give a history of trauma, but some are athletic individuals who play strenuous sports.

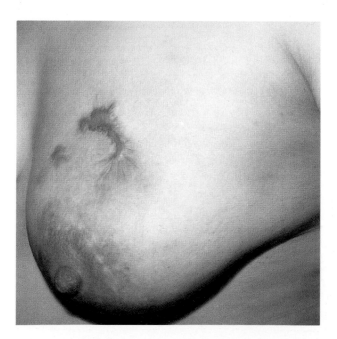

Figure 8.5
A case of a 28-year-old Chinese woman with scars of healed TB ulcers.

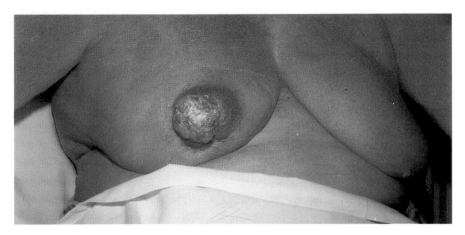

Figure 8.6

A 79-year-old woman with locally advanced but operable breast cancer.

Skin ulceration

Ulceration of the skin may occur in response to trauma, and sometimes can be self-inflicted. It may also be seen as part of the process of chronic infection in patients with tuberculosis. Once rare in Britain, it is now being seen more frequently among recently arrived immigrants.

The main cause of skin ulceration is a locally advanced breast cancer. Unfortunately there are still too many women who, for a variety of reasons, present with large ulcerated lesions. Sometimes they can be successfully

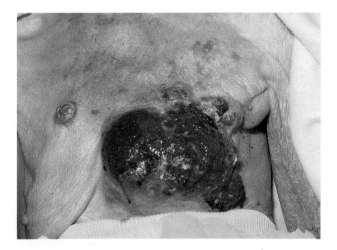

Figure 8.7

An 84-year-old woman with extensive skin ulceration. Disease was detected by the patient's daughter. The patient died 48 hours after admission.

palliated by surgery, which relieves them of the need for frequent dressings and stops the unpleasant smell from anaerobic bacterial infection.

Skin infiltration

Prior to the onset of ulceration, malignant cells may invade the dermis and epidermis to produce a yellow plaque which subsequently becomes red before ulcerating. Although skin infiltration is deemed to be an indicator of inoperability, if localised the skin may be excised with the cancer and mastectomy may be feasible. Skin infiltration is usually regarded as a contraindication for conservation therapy because of the skin-sparing nature of the radiotherapy that is used.

Postirraditional changes

Many of the skin changes that are sought when evaluating a suspicious lump

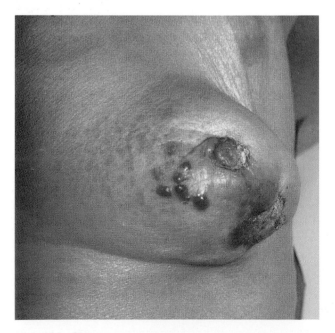

Figure 8.8

A case of locally advanced breast cancer showing skin ulceration, infiltration, and skin nodular metastases.

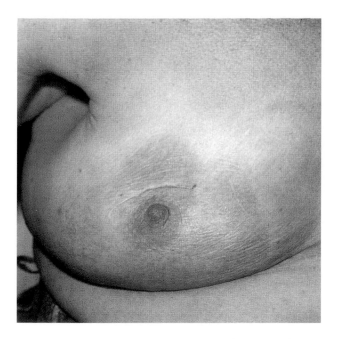

Figure 8.9
Radiotherapy can lead to skin hyperpigmentation.

will occur as consequences of breast irradiation. Thus, during treatment, skin erythema is common and this may be followed by pigmentation of the skin and depigmentation of the nipple/areola.

Additionally, radiotherapy can produce lymphatic obstruction with *peau*

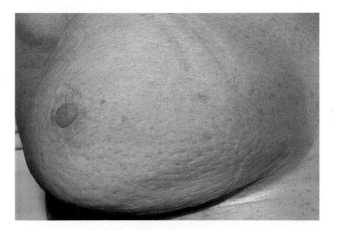

Figure 8.10
Postirradiation erythema and *peau d'orange*.

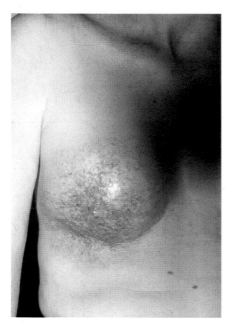

Figure 8.11

A case of postirradiation skin fibrosis and marbling of the right breast. The patient suffered from recurrent skin ulceration. She was eventually treated by mastectomy and breast reconstruction.

d'orange of the irradiated skin. Late results of radiation include skin marbling and telangiectases, often associated with breast fibrosis, particularly at the site of a radiation boost.

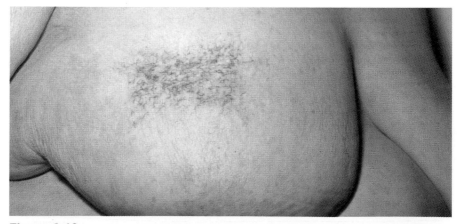

Figure 8.12
A case of postirradiation telangiectasia.

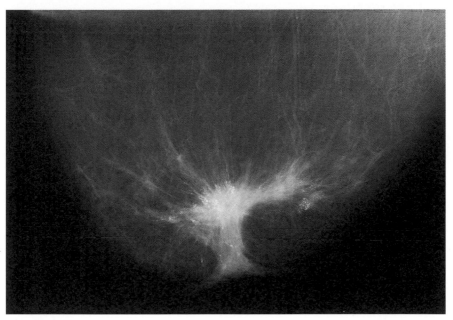

Figure 8.13

A mammogram of extensive breast cancer. Note the skin thickening and the honeycomb appearances indicative of *peau d'orange.*

Skin oedema on mammograms

One of the signs suggestive of malignancy on a mammogram is thickening of the breast skin. When this is seen overlying an opacity it is likely that the lesion is malignant. However, if the patient has already had a cancer, treated by conservation therapy, there may be distortion of the breast tissue with overlying skin oedema, both of which result from postradiation fibrosis, not recurrence of diseases. Thus, when ordering follow-up mammograms in patients who have been treated for breast cancer, it is most important that the radiologist is given a full history and details of treatment.

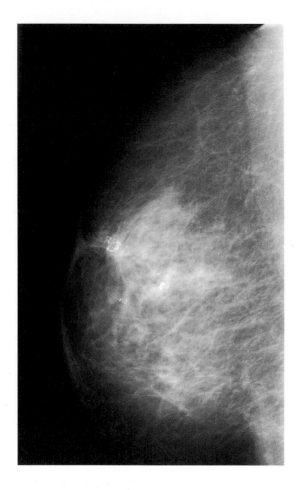

Figure 8.14

A follow-up mammography of a previously erradicated breast. Note the skin thickening of the inferior part and the honeycomb appearances, indicative of skin oedema.

KEY POINTS

- Examination in a good light is necessary to detect subtle skin changes.
- *Peau d'orange* may be a sinister sign but also is a consequence of irradiation.
- Skin tethering can be a sign of cancer but in the absence of a lump may be due to thrombophlebitis.
- Ulceration of the skin may be infective or factitious but malignancy must be considered.

9
BREAST CANCER

The fear of women who have found a breast lump and the object of breast assessment is to make a diagnosis of breast cancer. Careful examination which can convince a patient that she has no serious pathology is the cornerstone of assessment. Nevertheless, a few patients will have a lump which will prove eventually to be malignant. If this is suspected by the examiner, it is best that the potential diagnosis is shared with the patient. This can serve to minimise the impact of a diagnosis of malignancy. Allowing the patient to come to terms with the diagnosis is an important part of the management of breast cancer.

The lump

Breast cancer is characteristically a hard irregular lump which is usually not painful. There may be associated signs of invasiveness such as skin tethering or puckering on movement. Additionally, lumps close to the nipple may cause inversion, or a blood-stained or serous discharge.

The lump itself may show evidence of deep tethering or fixation, confirmed by asking the patient to tense the pectoralis major muscle by pushing the arms in towards the hips. Occasionally, there is Paget's disease of the nipple associated with the lump, and there may be a blood-stained or serous discharge from the nipple.

Measurement

Once a clinical diagnosis of breast cancer has been made, it is important to record accurately the dimensions of the lump and any other associated clinical signs. The reason for this is that diagnostic tests such as core needle biopsy or FNAC may lead to an alteration in the clinical signs because of haematoma formation or merely surgical trauma.

Measurements should be made with calipers, rather than a tape measure or ruler. Descriptive terms such as 'walnut-sized', 'grape' and 'grain of rice' are inadequate, and should be replaced with dimensions in centimetres.

The axilla

Examination of the axilla can be very difficult, and this can be compounded if the suspensory ligament of the axilla is tensed by the arm being in an abducted position. Thus it is essential that palpation is conducted while supporting the patient's arm by her side.

Only after this manoeuvre can the apex of the axilla be palpated. If nodes are present they should be measured and a note made of their mobility or attachment. Particularly serious are matted nodes which are usually indicative of extensive axillary nodal involvement, and are regarded by some as a sign of inoperability.

The neck

Although the neck should be inspected from the front, examination should be performed from behind the patient so that both anterior and posterior triangles of the neck can be thoroughly palpated and any nodes present can be measured. It is relatively unusual for patients with early breast cancer to have supraclavicular nodal involvement at the time of presentation, but individuals with locally advanced disease may display evidence of cervical node metastases. If a suspicious node is found and a decision made to perform FNAC, this should be carried out by an experienced operator, to minimise the risk of damage to surrounding structures.

The chest

After examining the neck the posterior aspect of the thorax can be inspected for evidence of skin changes and the chest can be percussed to exclude the stony dullness of a pleural effusion in a patient with stage III or IV disease.

Additionally, the vertebral column can be inspected for evidence of scoliosis or a step suggestive of vertebral collapse. The spine can be gently percussed to detect any localised bone tenderness.

The abdomen

After the patient has been asked to lie flat, the abdomen is inspected for signs of ascites. In the absence of symptoms suggestive of intra-abdominal

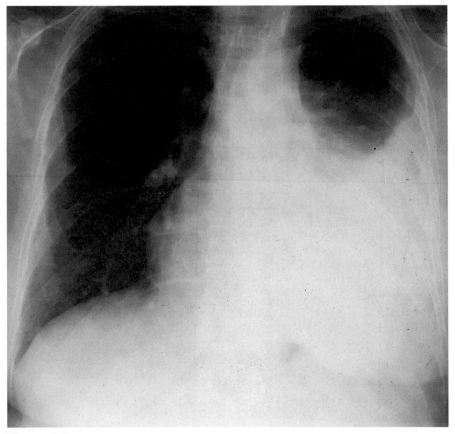

Figure 9.1
A chest X-ray showing left-sided pleural effusion.

pathology, a gentle palpation is performed, checking in particular for evidence of hepatomegaly. If the liver is palpable the extent should be recorded as the distance in centimetres from liver edge to the costal margin in the mid-clavicular line.

Locally advanced breast cancer

Unfortunately there are still too many women who present with fungating or ulcerated breast cancers because they have delayed seeing a doctor for a variety of reasons. Such patients are often guilt-ridden and this can be compounded if the doctor adopts an aggressive stance – 'You've been very silly'. These patients have incurable disease and their subsequent quality of life will be diminished greatly if they are made to feel guilty.

In the short term those with fungating lesions can be helped by metronidazole, which will diminish the smell arising from anaerobic secondary infection. Sometimes it is possible to carry out a surgical procedure to rid them of the fungating or ulcerated lesion so that they no longer need daily dressings.

It is most important that all lesions are measured and, when possible, photographed in order that responses to treatment can be monitored. Unless there are life-threatening metastases in liver, lung, or brain, it is customary to start with endocrine therapy which would usually be tamoxifen since the majority of these patients are postmenopausal.

Some will have symptomatic pleural effusions and palliation can be achieved in the majority by performing a talc pleurodesis. This is usually performed under general anaesthesia, but is possible using local anaesthetic.

KEY POINTS

- If breast cancer is suspected all relevant clinical signs should be recorded and measured.
- Such patients need urgent referral.
- Patients who present with advanced breast cancer need sympathy not admonition.

10
BREAST CANCER FOLLOW UP

There has been a considerable amount of discussion on the most appropriate follow up for patients who have been treated for breast cancer. This relates to the nature of follow-up tests, intensity, and timing, and whether this should be the responsibility of the hospital or the GP.

The most important aspect is the attitude of the patient; some are greatly reassured by hospital follow up, others spend the days before their visit in great trepidation and may not be reassured after seeing a different doctor at each clinic appointment. As an additional complication, patients who have been treated by mastectomy may be relatively easy to assess, whereas those who have had breast conservation therapy may have clinical signs which are difficult to interpret.

General health

Patients who are feeling well are very unlikely to have systemic relapse of breast cancer but local recurrence is usually not associated with general symptoms. If primary treatment has been effective there will be a low probability of local recurrence and, similarly, appropriate adjuvant therapy will substantially reduce the risk of both locoregional and distant relapse. Despite this, some patients will relapse and the commonest site is bone. Thus symptoms of localised bone pain or aching need evaluation by either radioisotopic bone scan or skeletal X-rays.

Similarly, breast cancer patients with shortness of breath or symptoms of pleurisy need a chest X-ray to exclude pulmonary or pleural metastases. Nevertheless, it should be remembered that breast cancer is not a protection against viral or degenerative diseases and the majority of symptomatic breast cancer cases will have a benign cause for their problems.

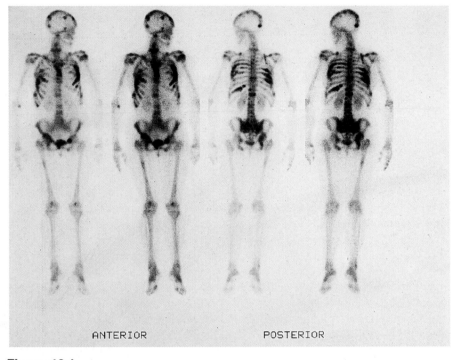

ANTERIOR   POSTERIOR

Figure 10.1

A 45-year-old woman, previously treated for breast cancer, presented with constant back pain. An isotopic bone scan showed widespread bone metastases.

Frequency of follow up is variable and may depend upon the clinician's view of the patient's prognosis. In most breast clinics patients are seen every 3 months for the first 3 years, 6 monthly for the next 2 years, and then annually once they reach their fifth anniversary after diagnosis.

Mastectomy scar

The scar should be inspected with the arm at the side and then again after abducting the shoulder. This gives a better view and also confirms that the patient has regained full shoulder mobility postoperatively. The scar and surrounding tissue are then palpated and note taken of any nodules, the dimensions of which are recorded.

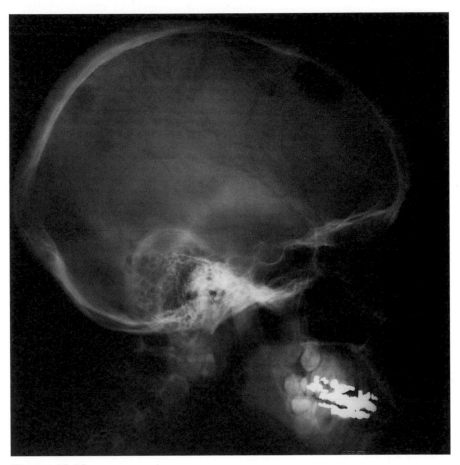

Figure 10.1A
Skull X-ray as part of a skeletal survey of a 50-year-old woman who had previously treated breast cancer. Lytic bone metastases can be seen on the X-ray.

FNAC can be taken of any suspicious nodules. Sometimes it is necessary to carry out an excision biopsy under local anesthetic. Single skin recurrences can be associated with a good prognosis when treated by excision and postoperative irradiation. Multiple skin recurrences carry a bad prognosis and these patients should be considered for some form of systemic adjuvant therapy.

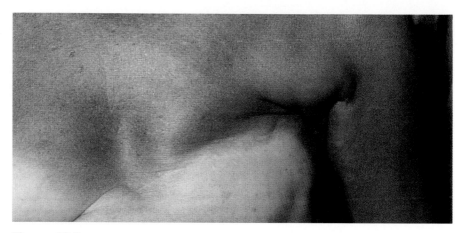

Figure 10.2
A well-healed mastectomy scar with no evidence of relapse.

Axilla and neck

After the chest wall has been checked, the axilla is palpated while supporting the patient's arm by her side so that it can be carefully assessed. Following this, the patient's neck is inspected and then examined from behind, measuring any palpable lesions and noting whether these are mobile or fixed. Since the patient is now sitting up, the chest can be percussed at the bases to detect a pleural effusion.

Contralateral breast

Approximately 1% of breast cancer patients will develop a contralateral mammary malignancy every year, this risk remains constant and does not diminish as time elapses after first treatment. It is for this reason that contralateral breast examination is an essential part of the follow-up of breast cancer cases. Palpation should be performed with the patient lying down and also turned half on her side to facilitate examination of the upper outer quadrant and axillary tail.

General examination

It is customary to palpate the abdomen, and in particular to determine whether there is hepatomegaly. It is very unusual for a breast cancer patient to have liver enlargement due to metastases without some symptoms such as epigastric discomfort or pain, weight loss, or nausea.

Should the patient give specific symptoms the examiner can then concentrate on examining that system, such as the CNS in patients with headache, weakness, or behavioural change. Localised bone pain is suspicious of metastatic disease, but persistent backache in a breast cancer patient is also an indication for skeletal imaging.

Breast conservation

Evaluation of the conserved breast can be very difficult and even the most experienced clinicians may be wrong sometimes. Assessment can be made even more difficult in patients who have had a boost to the excision site, either externally or by implant.

If there is doubt in the mind of the examiner, the advice of the most experienced surgeon or radiotherapist should be sought. Probably the most important sign is a documented increase in the extent of a region of induration.

Palpation of excision site

The biopsy scar is inspected and the patient asked whether she has noticed any change, particularly if the nipple is becoming inverted. This is almost never the result of postradiational scarring but usually a sign that local recurrence has occurred.

It is common for there to be induration at the site of excision, particularly after a local boost. The dimensions of the induration should be measured and recorded. If the induration has been noted previously and has not changed, no action need be taken.

However, should there be an increase in extent, FNAC should be performed. It is important that the cytology is reviewed by an experienced cytopathologist, because atypical cells may be present as a result of radiation changes and these should not be taken to indicate recurrence. Additionally, it is essential that the cytopathologist is told that the breast has been irradiated previously. Under these circumstances, a core needle biopsy may be carried out in addition to FNAC.

Measurement of breast compression

As a result of breast irradiation, skin oedema may be present and this occurs more frequently in patients who have had an axillary clearance. This *peau d'orange* may be associated with generalised induration of the underlying breast tissue. To measure the extent of breast induration, a tape measure is placed horizontally on the breast with the 5 cm mark on the nipple. A finger and thumb are placed 10 cm apart and then the breast tissue compressed.

The measurement between thumb and finger after compression is recorded and compared with the same compression on the untreated breast. As time elapses after breast irradiation, so the compression measurement on the affected side should diminish and come closer to the untreated side.

Lymphoedema

The majority of patients who have had an axillary clearance will not develop lymphoedema of the ipsilateral arm. However, if the patient has axillary irradiation and develops a recurrence at that site so that a subsequent surgical clearance is necessary, there is a high risk of arm swelling.

Lymphoedema is measured by recording the arm circumference 15 cm above the olecranon process and 10 cm below. This is compared with the same measurements on the untreated side. These dimensions form the basis of determining the presence of lymphoedema, remembering that the dominant arm may be 1–2 cm greater in circumference than the non-dominant side. These simple measurements can serve also to monitor response to decompression therapy.

Follow-up tests

It has been found that most of the follow-up investigations used in patients with early breast cancer do not serve any useful purpose from the point of

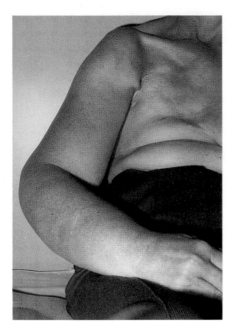

Figure 10.3

Lymphoedema of the right arm
following radical mastectomy.

view of an asymptomatic patient. Measurements of so-called tumour markers
do not give useful information. Similarly, routine bone scans may pick up
asymptomatic bone metastases but this gives only a few months of lead time
with no benefit to the patient from instigating earlier therapy because the
disease is incurable.

The one exception is the use of follow-up mammography, on an annual or
biennial basis. This may detect impalpable and potentially curable disease in
the contralateral breast. Additionally, early relapse in the conserved breast
may be identified. However, it can be difficult to distinguish radiologically
between postradiation/surgical changes and the fibrosis associated with
recurrence of disease.

Under these circumstances an MRI scan with enhancement using Gd-
DTPA may be useful in the detection of early relapse. An MRI scan is taken of
the breast and then the scan repeated after injection of the enhancing agent.
Areas of relapse show up as white regions on the postinjection films which
were not present on the baseline views.

However, this may bring new problems when there is no clinical or
mammographic evidence of recurrence but a suspicious area on the MRI
scan. Localisation of the suspicious lesion can be achieved using a non-
ferrous marker such as tungsten and inserting this under MRI control.

There will be increasing pressure for general practitioners to follow up their

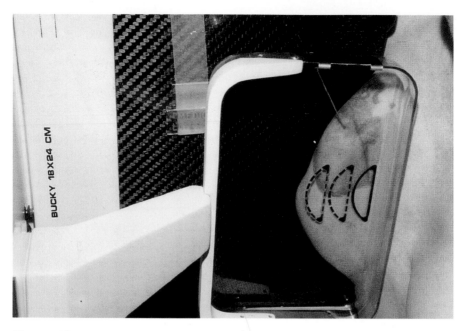

Figure 10.4
Needle localisation of impalpable breast pathology.

breast cancer patients. Although this is less problematical for those who have undergone mastectomy, the evaluation of the irradiated breast can be very difficult. Patients with equivocal or apparently progressive fibrosis should be referred for a specialist opinion.

KEY POINTS

- There is no evidence that intensive hospital follow up benefits patients who have been treated for early breast cancer.
- Patients who have had breast conservation may be difficult to assess and need specialist evaluation.
- The only routine follow-up investigation required is annual or biennial mammography.
- New symptoms, particularly of bone pain or breathlessness, need full investigation to exclude recurrence.

INDEX

Page numbers in **bold** refer to figures.

abdominal examination 57–8, 63
abscesses
  aspiration 45
  erythema 45
  lactation 27
  nipple inversion 27
  periareolar 13
  periductal mastitis 27
  smoking 20
accessory breast tissue 4, 9–10
adjuvant therapy 59, 61
amenorrhoea 9
anaerobic bacterial infections 50, 58
angina 24, 39
antibiotics 13, 15, 25
anxiety 1, 23
arthritis 39
ascites 57
Astley Cooper ligaments 3
asymmetry 4
atrophic scirrhous cancer 38
axilla
  accessory breast tissue 9–10
  bilateral mammary glands **5**
  cancer 56
  clearance 64, **65**
  examination 6, 56, 62
  lymphadenopathy 45
  nodes 56
  palpation 6–7, 56
  suspensory ligament 7, 56
axillary tail 6

backache 63
Bioptycut system **41–2**, 42
bone
  metastases **61**, 65
  pain 59, 63
  tenderness 57

breast bud, asynchronous growth 27
breast conservation therapy (BCT)
        see radiotherapy
breast lumps see lumps
breast pain 1, 22–6
  see also pain
  clinical examination 22
  cyclical 1, 22
  duct ectasia 22
  management algorithm 23–24, **23**
  nodularity 22
  non-cyclical 22
  older women 39
  postmenopausal 22, 23
  premenopausal 22
  severe 23–4
  treatment 25–6
  trigger point 24
bromocriptine 18, 25

carcinoma 55–8
  contralateral breast 62
  cystic **7**, 35
  erythema 45, **46**
  excision biopsy 37
  follow-up 59–66
  fungating lesions 58
  histological diagnosis 36–7
  local recurrence 59
  locally advanced 58
  lumps 55
  middle-aged women 36–7
  older women 38
  relapse 59
  typical appearance **41**
  ulceration 49–50, **49–50**, 58
  young women 30
chest examination 56–7
  percussion 62

X-rays **57**, 59
core needle biopsy 36, 40–42, **42**, 64
cysts
   aspiration 34–6
   excision biopsy 36
   fluid 34–5, **35**
   mammographic appearance **34**
   middle-aged women 32, 34–6
   Montgomery's gland 9
   multiple 34
   older women 39
   papillary carcinoma 39
   recurrent 36
   treatment 34–5
   young women 27
cytology 63–4

D2 dopamine agonists 18
danazol 25
duct ectasia
   erythema 45
   nipple discharge 18–20
   nipple indrawing 5
   nipple inversion 10, 11
   older women 39
   pain 22
ductal carcinoma in situ (DCIS)
   nipple discharge 18, 21
   older women 40
   Paget's disease 11–12
ducts
   dilatation/shortening 5
   excision (microdochectomy) 17, 20–21
   multiple 20
   papilloma 18, 20–21

early diagnosis 1
eczema 1
   areola **12**, 13
   nipple 5, 11
erythema 45, **46**
evening primrose oil (EPO) 25

family history 32
fat necrosis **43**, 47
fibroadenomas
   calcifying 40

giant 28, **29**
   growth spurt during lactation 29
   macrocalcification **33**, 34
   middle-aged women 33–4
   older women 39–40
   young women 27, 28
fibroadenosis *see* nodularity, localised
fibrocystic disease 18
fibrosis
   postradiation 53
   recurrent cancer 65–6
fine needle aspiration cytology (FNAC)
   induration at excision site 63
   infiltrating lobular carcinoma 36
   lumps 28
   middle-aged women 33
   neck nodes 56
   older women 43–4
   recurrent nodules 61
   young women 28
fistulas, mammillary 13–15
flucloxacillin 45
frozen sections 37, 43
fungating lesions 58

galactocoeles (milk cysts) 27, 29, **30**
galactorrhoea 8, 18, **19**
galactorrhoea-amenorrhoea
      syndrome 9
gall stones 24
goserelin 26
GPs 36, 65–6

hepatomegaly 58, 63
hiatus hernia 24
hirsutism 8
history taking 1
hormone replacement therapy
      22, 32, 39
hyperprolactinaemia 8, 18

induration 63, 64
infiltrating lobular carcinoma 36
inflammatory carcinoma 45
invasive carcinoma
   nipple discharge 18, 21
   Paget's disease 11, 12

involution
  post-lactation 18
  postmenopausal 39

lactation
  abscesses 27
  milk cyst (galactocoele) 27, 29, **30**
  normal 18
lateral thoracic vein
      thrombophlebitis (Mondor's
      syndrome) 3, **4**, 47–8, **48**
lumps
  excision biopsy 30, 33
  fine needle aspiration cytology 28
  lactation 29
  malignant 55
  measurement 55–6
  middle-aged women 32–7
  older women 38–44
  patient pointing to 5, **6**
  peau d'orange 45
  ultrasound 28
  young women 27–31
lymphoedema 64, **65**

mammillary fistula 13–15, 20
mammography 32, 33, 40, 65
  cysts 36
  extensive cancer **53**
  fat necrosis **43**
  nodularity 33, 39
  peau d'orange 53, **53–4**
mastalgia *see* breast pain
mastectomy
  lymphoedema 64, **65**
  modified radical 12–13
  older women 38–9
  Paget's disease 12–13
  radical 64, **65**
  scar 3–4, 60–61, **62**
metronidazole 58
microcalcification 40, **40**
microdochectomy 17, 20–21
middle-aged women 32–7
mock orange syndrome
      (*Philadelphus* spp.) 46–7, **46**
Mondor's syndrome 3, 4, 47–8, **48**

Montgomery's glands 4, 8, **8**
  cysts 9
MRI scan 65

National Breast Cancer Screening
      Programme 23
neck examination 56, 62
nipple-areolar complex **9**
  eczematous skin changes 1
  Paget's disease **12**
nipple discharge 16–21
  bloody 16–18, **17**
  cancer 55
  clear 20–21, **20**
  history taking 1
  inverted nipples 10–11
  management algorithm 16–18, **16**
  milky (galactorrhoea) 8, 18, **19**
  physiological 8, 18
  serous/watery 17
  straw-coloured 21
  yellow 18–20, **19**
nipple inversion 1
  bilateral 11, **11**
  with discharge 10–11
  idiopathic 11
  local recurrence 63
  with mass 10
  older women 39
  postmenopausal 10
  unilateral 4, 10–11, **10**
nipples 8–15
  accessory 9–10
  depigmentation **14**, 15, 51
  eczema 5, 11
  hair 8
  indrawing 5
  inguinal 10
  inspection 4–5
  normal 8–9, **8**
  Paget's disease 5, 11–13, **12**
nodularity, localised (fibroadenosis) 45
  middle-aged women 33
  older women 39
  young women 27, 28

oestrogen 26

oestrogen receptor status 42
older women 38–44
oral contraceptives 18, 26, 32
osteochondritis 24

Paget's disease 5, 11–13, **12**, 55
pain
    bone 59, 63
    breast (mastalgia) *see* breast pain
    breast cancer 36
    duct ectasia 22
    extramammary 22, 24–5
    musculoskeletal 2, 24
    referred 22, 23
palpation 5–6
    contralateral breast 62
    excision site 63–4
papillary carcinoma 39
papilloma, intraduct 18, 20–21, **20**
papillomatosis, multiple 21
paraffin sections 37
peau d'orange 3, 45–6
    mammograms 53, **53–4**
    postirradiation 51–2, **51**, 64
pectoralis major muscle 55
periductal mastitis 18, 45
Philadelphus spp. 46–7, **46**
phyllodes tumour (cystosarcoma
       phylloides) 28
pituitary adenoma 8–9, 18
pleural effusion 56, **57**, 58, 62
pleural metastases 59
pleurisy 59
poorly differentiated (ductal grade III)
    cancers 28
positioning 2–4, **2–3**, 6, **7**
prepubertal girls 27
progesterone receptor status 42
pulmonary metastases 59

radiculitis 25
radioisotopic bone scan 59, **60**
radiotherapy 15, 43
    compression measurement 64
    depigmentation **14**, 15
    erythema 45, 51
    follow-up 63

hyperpigmentation **14**, 51, **51**
older women 38
postirradiational changes 50–52
skin recurrences 61

scoliosis 57
shortness of breath 59
skeletal X-rays 59
skin 45–54
    dimpling 3, **3**, **4**, **47**
    erythema 45
    fibrosis 52, **52**
    infiltration 50, **50**
    marbling 52, **52**
    nodular metastases **50**
    oedema see peau d'orange
    recurrences 61
    retained secretions **10**, 11
    telangiectases 52, **52**
    tethering 47, 55
    thickening 53, **53–4**
    ulceration 49–50, **48**
skull X-ray 61
smoking 13, 20, 45
staphylococcal infection 45
supraclavicular nodes 56
suspensory ligament 7, 56

talc pleurodesis 58
tamoxifen 25–6, 38, 58
telangiectases 52, **52**
Tietze's syndrome 24–5
Trucut biopsy 33, 40–42
tuberculosis ulcers **48**, 49
tumour markers 65

ultrasound 28
upper outer quadrant examination 6
urine testing sticks 16–17, **17**

vacutainer system **35**
vertebral column 57
vitamins 25
vitiligo 15

young women 27–31

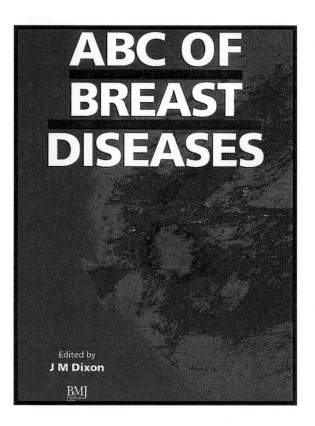

ABC of Breast Diseases

Edited by J M Dixon

Awarded Highly Commended - Royal Society of Medicine, Medical Book Awards

Breast conditions are so common that doctors in almost every specialty of medicine will be confronted at some time by a patient with a breast disorder. It is therefore vital that all doctors, especially general practitioners, have a knowledge of current methods of investigation and treatments for both benign and malignant breast diseases. This book, with the aid of full colour photographs and drawings, will help any doctor to make important diagnostic decisions to provide the best possible care for patients.

ISBN: 0 7279 0915 0

84 pages

Readership: general practitioners, practice nurses, medical students